10-Minute

other books in the same series

10-Minute Primer Chinese Kung Fu (Wushu)
Zhou Qingjie
ISBN 978 1 84819 213 3

10-Minute Primer Shaolin Quan
Zhou Qingjie
ISBN 978 1 84819 214 0

10-Minute Primer Tai Ji Quan
Zhou Qingjie
ISBN 978 1 84819 215 7

10-Minute Primer
QIGONG

Zhou Qingjie

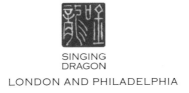

SINGING
DRAGON
LONDON AND PHILADELPHIA

This edition published in 2014
by Singing Dragon
an imprint of Jessica Kingsley Publishers
73 Collier Street
London N1 9BE, UK
and
400 Market Street, Suite 400
Philadelphia, PA 19106, USA

www.singingdragon.com

First edition published by Foreign Languages Press, Beijing, China, 2009

Library of Congress Cataloging in Publication Data
Zhou, Qingjie.
  10-minute primer qigong / Zhou Qingjie.
     pages cm.
  Originally published: Beijing : Foreign Languages Press, 2009.
  ISBN 978-1-84819-212-6 (alk. paper)
  1. Qi gong. I. Title. II. Title: Ten minute primer qigong.
  RA781.8.Z48 2014
  613.7'1489--dc23
                                        2013036910

British Library Cataloguing in Publication Data
A CIP catalogue record for this book is available from the British Library

ISBN 978 1 84819 212 6

Printed and bound in China

PRONUNCIATION GUIDE

气 qì—chee or *chi*
功 gōng—*gung* or *kung*

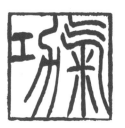

【CONTENTS】

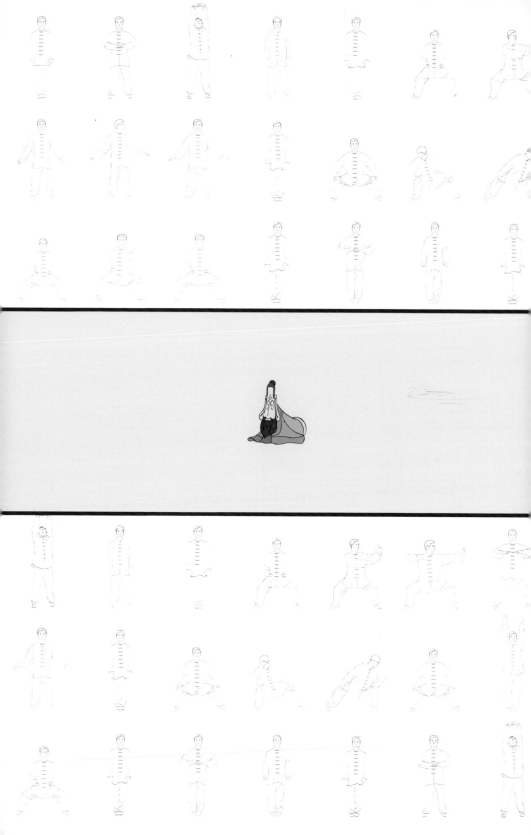

What is Qigong?

Qi

According to *The Contemporary Chinese Dictionary*, *qi* in Chinese medicine refers to the vital energy that enables all organs in the human body to function normally.

More than 2,200 years ago, the *Huangdi Neijing* or *Classic of Internal Medicine*, China's first comprehensive medical reference, included an elaborately detailed description of the function and purpose of *qi*. It said that *qi* is the chief source of all energy within the human body, and used *qi* as the common denominator to explain the body's physiological phenomena, the human spirit and

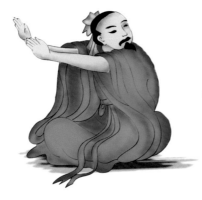

Illustrations of Physical and Breathing Exercises, each designed specifically for one of the traditional 24 Seasonal Divisions: Qigong exercise for the Beginning of Winter (around November 7 or 8)

consciousness, pathological changes, clinical diagnosis, and forms of treatment using acupuncture or drugs. It also gave names to more than 80 kinds of *qi* according to their different locations and functions, and made an extensive study of the important role of *qi* in the body.

Gong

Gong refers to skill and the attainment of skills. The *gong* in *qigong*, refers to the complete dedication to the attainment of a set goal.

Qigong

Qigong in ancient China was also called *tuna* (adjustment of breathing), *daoyin* (physical and breathing exercise), *zuochan* (sit in meditation) or *neigong* (internal exercise).

Qigong is defined as the skill of physical and mental training which integrates the functions of the body, breathing and the mind.

The benefits of *qigong* are many and varied. The *qigong* practitioner trains his mind, vital energy, and body in order to keep fit and prevent illness.

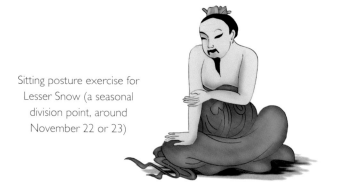

Sitting posture exercise for Lesser Snow (a seasonal division point, around November 22 or 23)

The objective of practicing *qigong* is to adjust the Yin and Yang balance in the body and to develop the potential ability to attain a very deep meditative state.

Make sure that *qi* is not interpreted solely as breathing and *qigong* is not understood simply as a breathing exercise. *Qigong* includes breathing exercises, but they are not the only or main objective.

Understanding Qigong

A world *qigong* conference was held in San Francisco in July 1999. It was attended by more than 500 scholars and masters from 16 countries engaged in *qigong* therapy and research. In view of its influence, former U.S. President Bill Clinton sent a letter of congratulation to the conference. The letter said that *Qigong*, an ancient art of health and medical science, has caught the attention of millions of people around the world. This traditional Chinese exercise, which stimulates the energy channels in the body, can contribute to people's overall physical fitness.

Now, please follow us passage by passage to open the ancient door to *qigong*.

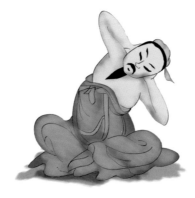

Exercise for
Autumn Equinox
(around September
22, 23 or 24)

The origin of qigong

Qigong originated from primitive man's efforts to protect health. Many of us have had the same experience: When we feel tired, we yawn, stretch or sit with our eyes closed. After a few moments, we're relaxed and more energized. It was exactly such conscious or unconscious behaviors that led to the formation of *qigong* as a means of fitness. Man first unconsciously and then consciously used *qigong* to keep fit and to prevent and cure illnesses. This was the origin of *qigong*.

Qigong in ancient times

Graves of the New Stone Age about 5,000 years ago were excavated by archaeologists in Qinghai Province in 1957. Among the relics unearthed was a colored ceramic basin painted with a lifelike dancing figure whose movements were related to ancient *qigong*.

A jade inscription of the Warring States Period now kept in the Tianjin Museum is the earliest and most significantly complete article describing *qigong* ever found. Scientists have dated it back to the end of the fifth century or the beginning of the fourth century BC. The inscription says: "In a cycle of breathing, a deep breath allows more air to be inhaled into the lungs. Expand the breath until it can go no deeper. When the air is exhaled, it is like the budding of the grass and trees, which continue to grow. Its exit route is opposite that of its intake, and it exits completely. When breathing, inhalation is like a heavenly secret, moving upward; exhalation is more of an earthly secret, moving down. One lives if he follows this truth, or dies if he acts against it."

The Sketch of *Daoyin* Physical and Breathing Exercises was a burial article unearthed from the No. 3 Tomb of the Han Dynasty at Mawangdui, Changsha, China, in December 1973. Buried in 168 BC, the colored diagram is painted on a

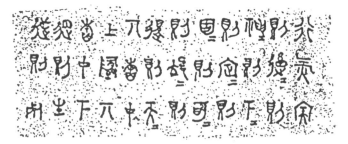

A jade inscription of the Warring States Period

piece of silk, showing men and women doing various *qigong* exercises. The diagram reflected the popularity of *qigong* at that time, and is therefore a highly treasured antiquity.

In the painting, more than 40 men and women are doing *daoyin* movements. They wear informal dress, and some men's torsos and feet are bare. They stand in four lines, with 11 people in each. Each is shown doing his or her individual exercises. Brief explanations of the exercises are written alongside most of the people. The movements and postures exhibited by these people are divided into three categories: breathing exercises, limb exercises, and exercises with weapons.

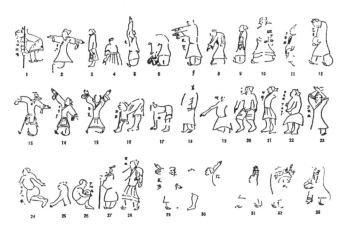

Sketch of Daoyin Physical and Breathing Exercises

Qigong concept of wholeness

The concept of wholeness is at the heart of Chinese
qigong. According to *qigong* beliefs, the parts of the
human body function in a coordinated way and influence
each other. At the same time, the human body and nature
are closely related.

In both theory and practice, Chinese *qigong* reflects the
concept of wholeness, which contains the idea that "man
and nature correspond to each other." Ancient *qigong*
masters used the concept of wholeness as their guiding
principle, and emphasized the close relationship between
man and his natural surroundings. *Qigong* regards the seven
emotions (joy, anger, melancholy, brooding, sorrow, fear
and shock) as the internal causes of disease, and the six
excesses (wind, cold, summer heat, humidity, dryness, and
fire) as the external causes of all ailments. While it stresses
that the internal factors play the dominant role, it also says
the external factors make an important contribution to
health and wellbeing, too.

The concept that man and nature are interrelated is an
important part of the idea of wholeness. *Qigong* practitioners
believe that the balance within the human body should be
in harmony with the external natural environment.

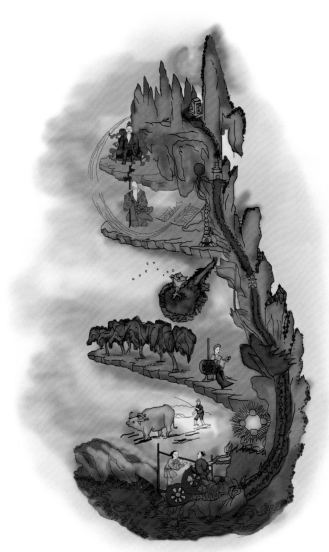

An imaginative view of the different
internal functions of the human body

One of the most important considerations when doing *qigong* exercises is the choice of time for doing them. The famous exercise of meridian *qi* circulation in *qigong* is based on the premise that there are 12 two-hour periods in a day, and both *qi* and blood in the twelve passages of the human body circulate in sequence in the given period. At this time, the physiological functions of each internal organ in each passage are most active, and doing an exercise suited for this particular period of time can help keep you physically fit and healthy.

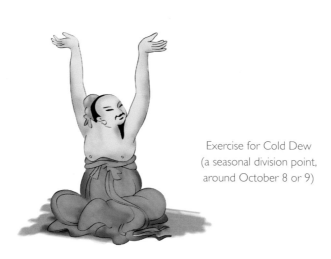

Exercise for Cold Dew
(a seasonal division point,
around October 8 or 9)

The 12 time divisions of a day* named after the 12 Terrestrial Branches during which the corresponding parts of the human body are considered most active and suitable for exercises:

The 12 two-hour periods of a day	Time	Internal organ
子 (zi)	23–1	Gallbladder
丑 (chou)	1–3	Liver
寅 (Yin)	3–5	Lung
卯 (mao)	5–7	Large intestine
辰 (chen)	7–9	Stomach
巳 (si)	9–11	Spleen
午 (wu)	11–13	Heart
未 (wei)	13–15	Small intestine
申 (shen)	15–17	Bladder
酉 (you)	17–19	Kidney
戌 (xu)	19–21	Pericardium
亥 (hai)	21–23	Sanjiao ("triple energizer" or 3 visceral cavities housing the internal organs)

(* In ancient China, people used these two-hour divisions to keep time.)

Theories of Yin and Yang
and the Five Elements

Yin and Yang and the five elements are at the heart
of Chinese *qigong*. They serve as the fundamental
guidelines for practicing *qigong* exercises. The Theory of Yin
and Yang is a philosophical concept. It holds that everything
on the earth has two aspects, Yin and Yang, and that the
opposites and unity inherent in Yin and Yang are the root
cause for the birth, change, and extinction of everything
in the universe. The world itself is the result of opposites,
unity, change and the development of Yin and Yang.

The Theory of the Five Elements originated from the
everyday activities of life of the people in ancient times.
People discovered that the five elements of metal, wood,
water, fire and earth were indispensable in daily life. The
theory maintained that all things in the world could be
grouped into five categories according to the Theory of
the Five Elements. And the interrelations and movements
determined the occurrence and development of all things.

The famous *qigong* exercise Liu Zi Jue or Six Sounds
Approach to Breathing Exercises is able to regulate the
internal organs to benefit physical fitness and cure illness.
This is achieved through the interrelation between the

phonetic sounds uttered during the exercise, the internal organs and the adjustment of breathing.

The Theory of Internal Organs and the Theory of Meridians

The Theory of Internal Organs is a model of the structure of the human body based on the Theories of Yin and Yang and the Five Elements. The five elements reflected in the internal organs are: heart (fire), liver (wood), spleen (earth), lung (metal) and kidney (water). The function of *qigong* in keeping in good health is to maintain the balance of the five internal organs.

The Theory of Meridians is a supplement to the Theory of Internal Organs. The meridians are internally related to the internal organs, and externally linked with the limbs. They connect the internal organs with the surface of the human body, and combine the internal organs to form an organic whole. Through the circulation of *qi* and blood, and the cultivation of Yin and Yang, they ensure that the functions of all parts of the human body are in harmony and relatively balanced.

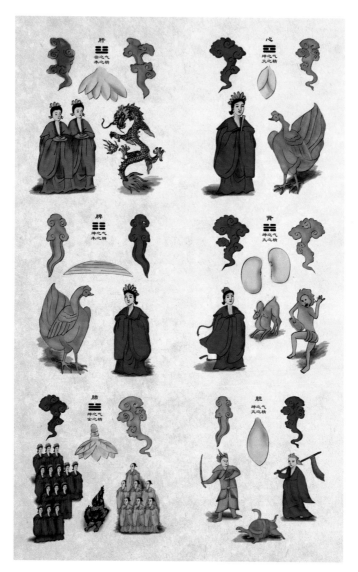

An ancient illustration of the human body's internal organs

The five internal organs are matched with five colors and five points of the compass or directions (which refer to the geographical positions which the qigong practitioners should face when they do exercises. The choice of direction is very important in the Chinese traditional qigong exercise!):

Metal — lung — west — white
Wood — liver — east — green
Water — kidney — north — black
Fire — heart — south — red
Earth — spleen — center — yellow

Jing, qi, shen or body essence, vital energy, and state of mind

Ancient *qigong* masters believed that there were three treasures in heaven: the sun, the moon and the stars; there were three treasures on earth: water, fire and wind; and that man had three treasures: *jing*, *qi* and *shen*. They regarded *jing*, *qi* and *shen* as the three most treasured parts of the human body, and as the only substances that are indispensable in life and necessary for the body to function properly.

Jing or body essence refers to every substance that is useful and that nourishes the human body; it is the material foundation of the human body.

Qi or vital energy refers to an abstruse substance that sustains the human body or the function of the internal organs.

Shen or state of mind governs the activities of the human body. Though invisible, it is the driving force for all the activities of life.

Jing, *qi* and *shen* each have their own characteristics, but they are inseparable. *Jing* is the source of *shen*. If there is *jing*, there is *shen*. Therefore, once *jing* is accumulated, it can make *shen* complete. *Jing* is also inhabited by *qi*. *Jing*, *qi* and *shen* are a trinity, always staying together. If one exists, they all exist. And if one dies, they all die.

The training and maintenance of *jing*, *qi* and *shen* in *qigong* can make the practitioners vigorous and physically strong.

The dantian or "the elixir field" is located in the pelvic region about the width of three fingers directly below the navel. The dantian is the place where the qi and the body's energy are concentrated. It represents a very important place in qigong.

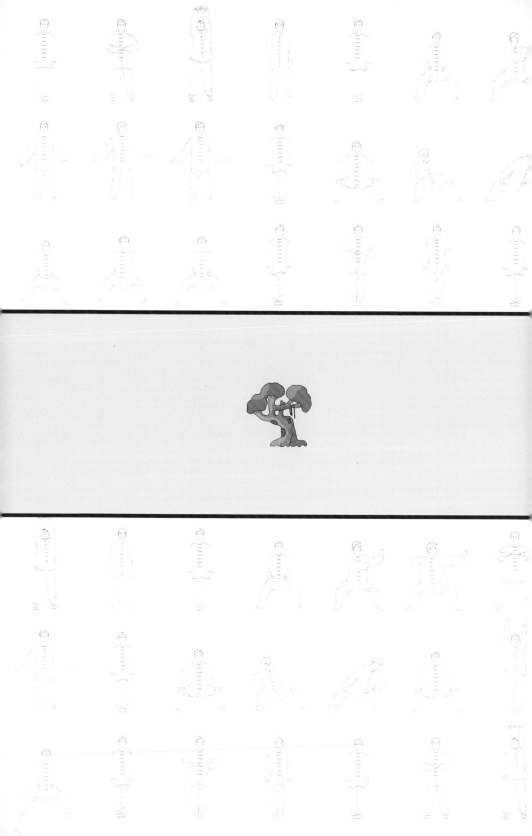

Qigong and Health

Benefits of the systematic practice of qigong

Prevent illness

There is an old saying in Chinese medicine: "A good doctor prevents a disease rather than merely curing it." This means that the best doctors are not those who have the necessary skills to perform surgery but those who know how to kill diseases before people contract them. This concept is one of the first benefits that can be received from *qigong*.

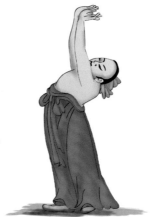

Exercise for Grain in Ear
(a seasonal division point,
around June 5, 6 or 7)

Improve the state of mind

Qigong is an exercise that requires the use of your thinking, breathing and body to improve your health and state of mind. The slow, fluid *qigong* movements will create a feeling of calm and relaxation that will penetrate into many aspects of life. The obvious effects of *qigong* are the ability to concentrate more fully and a heightened ability to ignore distractions. There is no doubt that *qigong* has exceptional health benefits and also can have a positive effect on work and study.

Improve the cardiovascular system and respiratory system

The most noticeable physiological change in the course of practicing *qigong* is the motion of the respiratory organs. *Qigong* has special requirements for breathing: the breathing cycle is longer, the rhythm is slow, the scope is deep, and the breaths are even and soft. Improvement of the function of the respiratory system will have a corresponding impact on the nervous system; this in turn affects the cardiovascular system so that the contraction and expansion of the heart and blood vessels will be improved. The most direct effect is that the lowered heart rate will also lower blood pressure. Therefore, *qigong* is an excellent choice for the cure of cardiovascular disease.

Improve the digestive system

As abdominal breathing is used in the course of practicing *qigong*, it helps to regularly massage the organs and cavities of the human body. It also promotes the involuntary muscle contractions of the stomach and intestines, reduces the stagnation of the blood in the abdominal cavity, improves the regulation of hormones, and balances the digestive functions. Therefore, *qigong* will usually increase your appetite. All of these effects can help to cure illness.

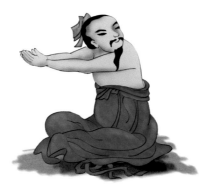

Exercise for Spring
Equinox (around
March 20 or 21)

People who are especially skilled at *qigong* can use their mind to regulate their nervous system and internal organs. Some have the ability to produce an unusual electrical or magnetic effect around them, thus creating a change in the magnetic field around the body and helping to produce or receive electromagnetic waves. People who have practiced *qigong* for a long time and reached a certain level of expertise are more sensitive to magnetic signals than other people. It is believed that people who practice *qigong* for years have increased senses of warmth or cold when facing north or south with their eyes covered. Some long-time practitioners can accurately determine directions within magnetic fields.

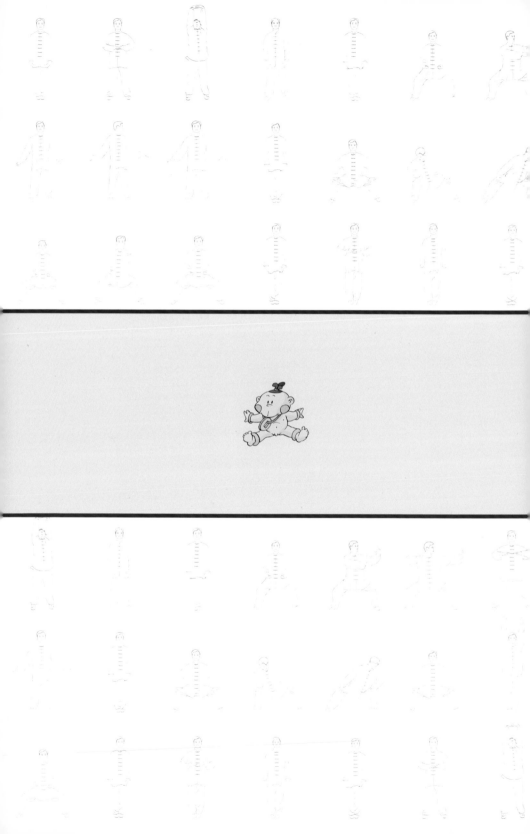

Qigong Postures

The posture used when practicing *qigong* is also referred to as body adjustment: the skill of training the body to adapt to a specific form. Good posture is the first step in practicing *qigong*. A natural and relaxed posture is the prerequisite for doing *qigong* breathing properly and inducing a calm state of mind. Different postures have different physiological characteristics. The common postures include the standing posture, sitting posture and lying posture.

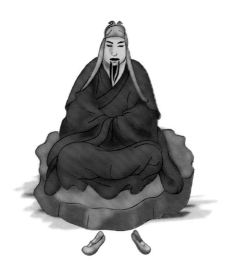

An ancient posture of sitting cross-legged

Standing posture

The standing posture is the basic posture for the stake-standing exercise.

Ball-holding posture

Keep the feet apart to the width of the shoulders, step slightly inward, knees slightly bent, chest drawn in, both arms raised with the hands to the shoulder level, and elbows lower than the shoulders. Keep the hands apart, with the distance between as wide as the length of two hands, arms curved into the shape of a semi-circle, as if holding a round balloon. Keep the fingers apart, slightly bent. Keep the head upright, eyes and mouth slightly closed, and lower jaw slightly drawn in. Be fully relaxed after the posture is ready. The ball-holding posture is also called the three-circle posture, i.e. the legs, arms and hands all bend to form a circular posture.

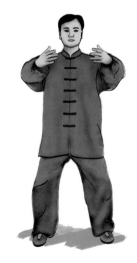

Sitting posture

The sitting posture is the most common posture used for doing the static *qigong* exercise.

Sitting upright

Sit upright on a square stool or a hard chair, feet apart on the ground to the width of the shoulders, trunk forming a 90 degree angle with the thighs and then with the calves. Put the hands on the knees or lightly clench fists on the lower abdomen, chin slightly drawn, shoulders down, chest drawn in, mouth and eyes slightly closed, the tip of the tongue touching the upper jaw, and the body naturally relaxed.

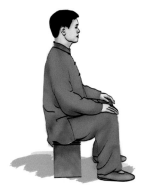

Sitting cross-legged

Sitting crossed-legged is the most appropriate posture for doing static *qigong* exercise. Sit on a bed or low square stool specially made for this purpose. A cushion should be put on it. The cushion should be thicker if you sit on the floor or ground. There are three postures for sitting cross-legged: sitting naturally cross-legged, sitting with one leg crossed, and sitting with both legs crossed.

Sitting naturally cross-legged: Sit upright on a cushion with the legs crossed, either the left leg on the right or the right leg on the left, both hands down on the thighs or knees, or clasped lightly before the lower abdomen.

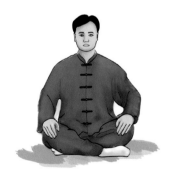

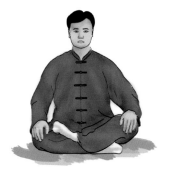

Sitting with single leg crossed: Sit upright on a cushion, right leg on the left leg or vice versa, both hands down on the thighs or knees, or clasped lightly before the lower abdomen.

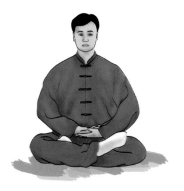

Sitting with both legs crossed: Sit upright on a cushion. First put the left foot or right foot on the opposite leg and then do the same with the other foot, keep the soles of the feet up, both hands down on the thighs or knees, or clasped lightly before the lower abdomen.

Lying posture

When you practice *qigong* in the lying posture, use a pillow about 10 cm thick. The bed should not be too soft. If a wooden bed is used, a mat is needed.

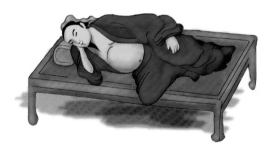

An ancient posture of lying on the side

Lying on the back

Lie flat on the bed, face up, head upright, and mouth and eyes slightly closed. The four limbs are naturally extended, arms at the sides. Keep both palms inside and lightly against the outer sides of the thighs, or bend the elbows with the hands placed on the lower abdomen (left hand under for men, right hand under for women).

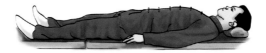

Lying on the side

Lie on the side on the bed, head flat on the pillow, upper part of the body straight, the leg above bent and put on the leg below, the hand above put on the hip and the hand below put on the pillow, palm up.

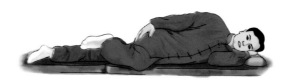

"The tip of the tongue touches the roof of the mouth" is the required position for the tongue when people do qigong. That is to say, the tongue should be placed naturally and lightly against the roof of the mouth. Qigong masters believe that this helps the practitioner fall into a meditative state and aids the smooth circulation of qi and blood in the meridian passages. Of course, not all qigong exercises require it. Some qigong exercises just require the practitioners to close their mouths and place the tongue naturally.

The saliva produced from the tip of the tongue touching the roof of the mouth can help to keep one's body immune from infection. It is interesting to note that the Chinese character 活 (live; alive) is a combination of 氵 for 水 (water) and 舌 (tongue).

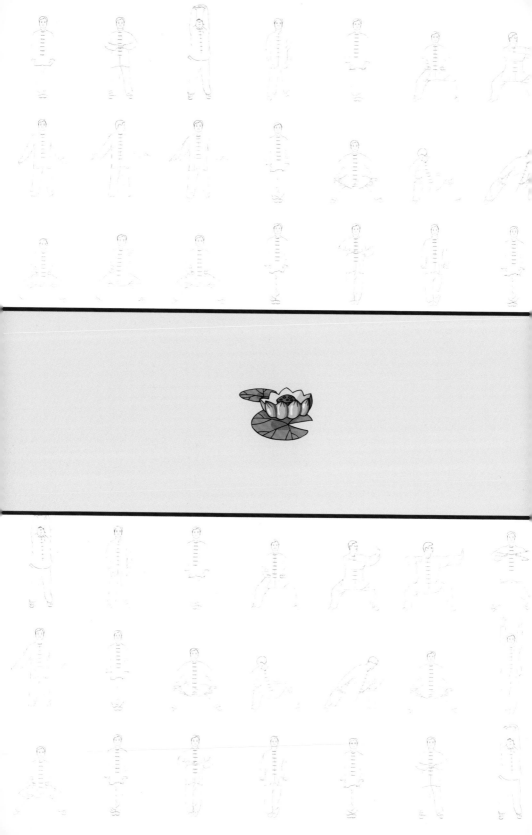

The Meditative State in Qigong

alling into a meditative state in *qigong* is also referred to as the adjustment of one's state of mind. It is the training of the mind. Adjustment of one's mind and a meditative state are the most fundamental skills used in practicing *qigong*. The effect of *qigong* exercise depends on the degree of the practitioner's meditative state; the more meditative you become, the better the effect. The meditative state achieved during exercise calls for you to have no distracting thoughts; your mind is focused either on the *dantian* or on your breathing. As one gets better at reaching a meditative state, the body becomes less able to sense outside stimulation such as sound and light, and some practitioners can even achieve a feeling of weightlessness. There are five common methods for achieving the meditative state:

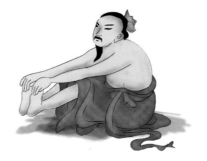

Exercise for Frost's Descent (a seasonal division point, around October 23 or 24)

Mental concentration

Mental concentration refers to intense concentration on one thing (such as on the *dantian*). When you concentrate, you should ignore distractions but you shouldn't have to work too hard at it; just focus naturally.

Focus on your breathing

This means that you concentrate on breathing; be aware of the changes in breathing and gently integrate your mind and vital energy in order to fall into the meditative state.

Exercise for Lesser Fullness of Grain (around May 20, 21 or 22)

Count while breathing

One breath equals one cycle of breathing in and out. When you do the exercise, silently count the number of breaths, from 1 to 10, from 10 to 100, until you hear nothing, see nothing, and think of nothing. In this way, you fall naturally into a meditative state.

Repeat words silently

The words repeated must be simple. The purpose of this is to use one thought to replace many distracting thoughts, and to use positive thinking to replace negative thoughts and thus fall into a meditative state. For example, the practitioner can just silently repeat the words "relax and be quiet."

Exercise for the Beginning of Summer (around May 5, 6 or 7)

Listen to your breathing

The practitioner listens to his own breathing until he hears nothing; by doing so he reaches the meditative state.

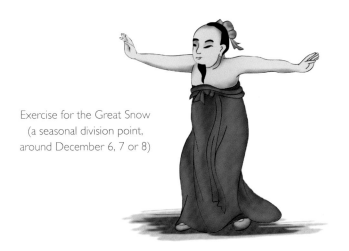

Exercise for the Great Snow
(a seasonal division point,
around December 6, 7 or 8)

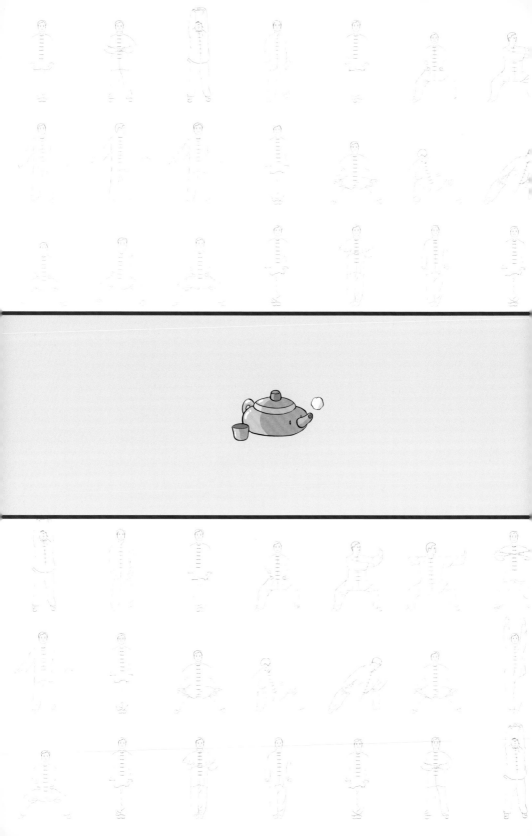

Breathing in Qigong

Breathing in *qigong* is also referred to as adjustment of breathing. It is one of the basic elements in the cultivation of *qi*. Proper breathing is an important link in falling into the meditative state. Through the training of breathing, the practitioner can regulate the tension of the sympathetic nerve and the parasympathetic nerve in the nervous system, expand the vital capacity of the lungs, promote normal breathing and improve blood circulation, massage the internal organs, aid digestion and absorption, keep in good health, and prevent and cure disease. The common breathing methods are as follows:

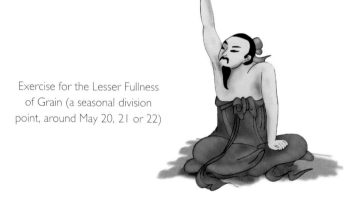

Exercise for the Lesser Fullness of Grain (a seasonal division point, around May 20, 21 or 22)

Thoracic breathing

Thoracic breathing is natural breathing. This is the normal physiological function everyone has and is not at all controlled by thought. The advantages of thoracic breathing are its softness and evenness; the disadvantage is that the individual breaths are not long enough.

Abdominal breathing

The main characteristic of abdominal breathing is that it is accompanied by the rise and fall of the abdomen. It is divided into normal abdominal breathing and counter-moving abdominal breathing.

Normal abdominal breathing means dilating the abdomen while inhaling and contracting it while exhaling. This is good for preventing and curing cardiovascular and cerebrovascular diseases.

Counter-moving abdominal breathing is just the opposite. It means contracting the abdomen while inhaling and dilating it while exhaling. This is good for preventing and curing diseases affecting the digestive system.

Transition from thoracic breathing to abdominal breathing is usually a transition to normal abdominal breathing. Counter-moving abdominal breathing involves more physical intensity and exercise and is more difficult than normal abdominal breathing. Special training is required under the guidance of a teacher.

It must be specially noted that whether doing normal abdominal breathing or counter-moving abdominal breathing, make sure to avoid bulging the abdomen intentionally when doing the exercise. The expansion and contraction of the abdomen mainly depends on the breathing. It is only supplementary.

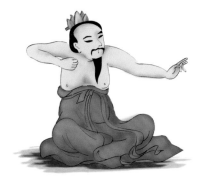

Exercise for the Pure
Brightness (around
April 4, 5 or 6)

Fetal breathing

Fetal breathing is a special breathing method used in *qigong*. This is in accordance with the Daoist idea of returning to nature and breathing softly, like a fetus taking air through the umbilical cord in its mother's womb. Fetal breathing is divided into two stages: navel breathing and body breathing.

Navel breathing is the equivalent of *dantian* breathing.

The biggest difference between body breathing and thoracic breathing or abdominal breathing is that the practitioner may feel as if the respiratory passage is no longer the mouth or nose. When body breathing is used in *qigong*, one feels that all pores on the body are opening and closing, the breath is coming and going through the pores, and there seems to be little breath moving through the mouth and nose.

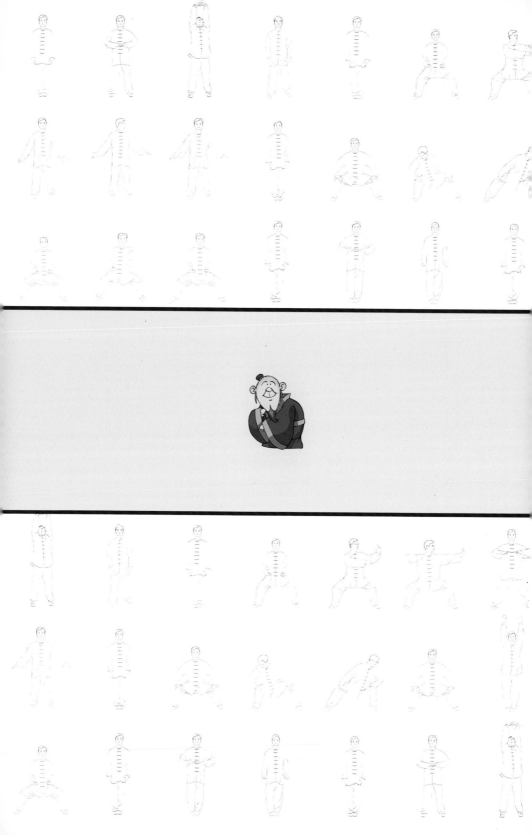

Baduanjin Qigong

Baduanjin *Qigong* originated in the Song Dynasty and has a history of more than 800 years. It is a kind of *qigong* mainly used for training body form (adjustment of posture). It places particular emphasis on the harmony between the limb and body movements, and breathing.

Baduanjin (Eight-Section Exercises) is specially designed for treating diseases and symptoms affecting the internal organs. Each section title clearly outlines the key points, function and purpose of the movement. The exercise consists of stretching, bending forward or backward, and rocking movements. These movements affect the "triple energizers"—the regions above the diaphragm, above the navel, and below the navel which include the heart, lungs, spleen, stomach, kidney and other organs. The exercise can help to prevent and cure many kinds of sickness and strain, including heartburn. It is good for developing muscles, increasing physical strength, improving the joints, strengthening the tendons and bones, helping digestion and regulating the nervous system.

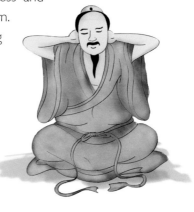

Jin (brocade) is name for a high-grade silk cloth in ancient China. Baduanjin, the name of the eight-section exercises, refers to its splendor and praises its effectiveness in curing illness and improving fitness.

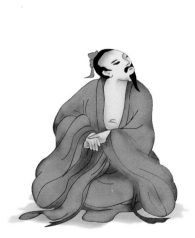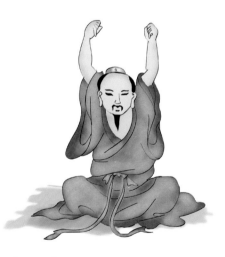

Ancient Baduanjin exercise

Starting position

Stand naturally with the feet together, arms naturally and loosely down by the sides, head and neck upright, chin slightly drawn in, eyes looking forward. Breathe naturally through the nose, and concentrate on the *dantian*.

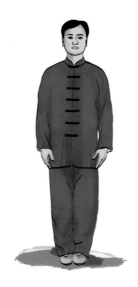

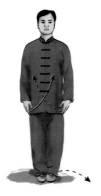

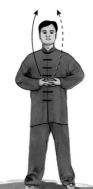

I. Holding the hands high with palms up to regulate the internal organs

Start by moving the left foot one step to the left, to the width of the shoulders. Cross the hands before the abdomen, palms up, and raise them upward along the mid-region of the body. Turn over the crossed hands (palms up) before the chest, and move up to right above the head, heels up, and eyes looking at the back of the hands. Do this exercise while inhaling.

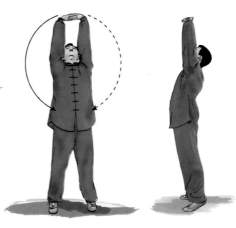

Loosen the crossed hands and lower them down by the sides. Place the heels down and return to the starting position, eyes gradually looking forward. Do this while exhaling.

Switch feet and do the same on the other side; repeat 6–8 times.

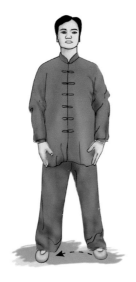 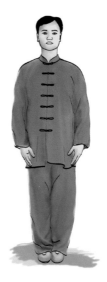

Key points

When the hands are raised upward, push the base of the palms upward with gentle force and stretch the back fully. When the heels are raised, straighten the knees to improve the body's balance.

Effect

Stretching the limbs and trunk has certain preventive and curative effects on cervical vertebra ailments, periarthritis, lumbago and back pain, and helps to correct poor posture. Raising the arms while breathing and increasing the breathing depth to supply more blood to the brain will help to alleviate fatigue.

The "triple energizer" is one of the vital organs, located between the chest and abdomen. Its main function is to remove obstacles from the water passage and stimulate the activity of *qi*. The triple energizer is divided into the upper energizer (above the diaphragm), the middle energizer (above the navel) and the lower energizer (below the navel).

It must be particularly noted that sufferers of periarthritis (inflammation of the joints around the shoulder) and dizziness should do these exercises as the ailment allows. One should avoid doing exercises if the body does not respond easily.

II. Posing as an archer shooting both left- and right-handed

Start by moving the left foot one step to the left, and bend both knees to squat in a horse stance (as though riding a horse). Make loose fists and place them by the hips.

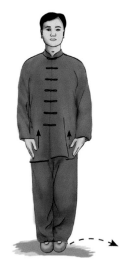
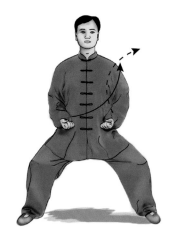

Lift the hands forward to chest level, clench the right fist with its thumb side up, and bend the elbow to the right as if drawing a bow as far as possible. At the same time, hold up the forefinger of the left hand, straighten the thumb outward to form the shape of "∟." Stretch the left elbow to the left as if to draw the bow to the arm length and push it upward to shoulder level, palm outward, eyes looking toward the left hand. Inhale while doing this exercise.

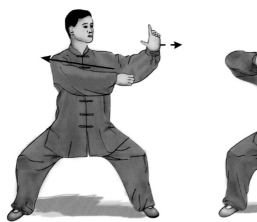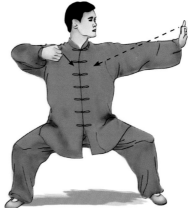

Straighten both legs and draw both hands back to the chest, press palms down and move them back to the hips. At the same time, move the left foot back to the starting position, eyes looking forward. Exhale while doing this.

Step out again; repeat 6–8 times.

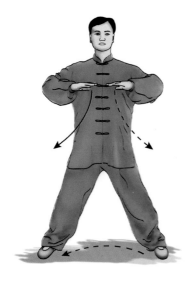
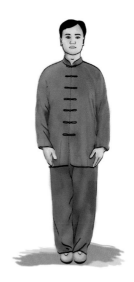

Key points

Pull the arms horizontally with equal force. Stretch the arms and expand the chest. Keep the head upright. While in the horse stance, keep the chest out and lower the waist; don't bend forward or backward.

Effect

While improving the functions of the heart and lungs, this can strengthen the muscles, bones and ligaments by stretching the arms, expanding the chest and turning the neck. The horse stance can increase leg strength.

III. Holding one arm aloft to regulate the functions of the spleen and stomach

Start by moving the left foot to the left, and draw arcs with both hands from the side of the body, moving them forward and inward, palms up and fingertips touching. After lifting both hands along the middle of the body up to the chest, move the left hand upward slowly, palm up, and with the fingers turned around 360 degrees counter-clockwise before stopping to point to the right, while moving it up to above the head till the arm is straight. At the same time, turn over the right hand, palm down, fingertips forward, and move the hands down to the side. The two hands vie with each other in pulling for power. Inhale while doing this exercise.

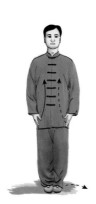 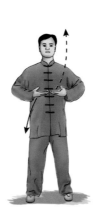 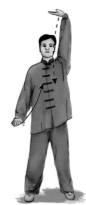

Move the left hand down slowly, turn the palm outward 360 degrees and then drop it down to the chest. At the same time, turn the right hand over and raise it to the chest. Turn the palms up, fingertips touching each other. Turn over both hands, palms down, and move them down slowly in an arc along the mid-region of the body, forward and outward before the abdomen, and draw them back to the sides. At the same time, move the left foot back to the starting position, eyes looking forward. Exhale while doing this exercise.

Switch feet and do the same movements on the other side; repeat 6–8 times.

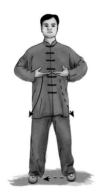 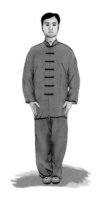

Key points

Move the palms up and down alternately and stretch them fully, straighten the arms, keep the chest out and straighten the back.

Effect

Shrink the abdominal cavity, stretch and relax the back and abdomen, and massage the organs in the abdominal cavity. This promotes the natural action of the intestines and stomach, and improves digestion.

Note

It must be particularly noted that people with periarthritis should do this exercise with caution.

IV. Looking backwards to prevent sickness and strain

Start by moving the left foot one step to the left to the width of the shoulders; at the same time move the hands apart to both sides to form an angle of about 45 degrees, palms back. Inhale while doing this exercise.

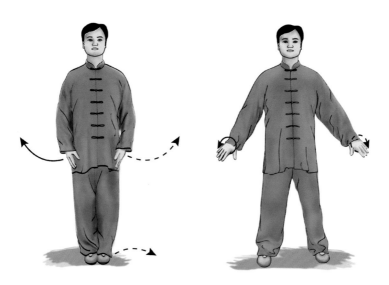

Keep the upper part of the body and the lower limbs still, turn the head to the left and look back. At the same time, turn the hands over, palms out. Exhale while doing this.

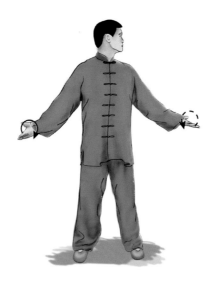

Turn the head back to the original position, and at the same time turn the hands over, palms down, eyes looking forward. Inhale while doing this.

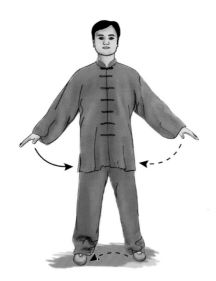

Move the hands back to the sides, and at the same time move back the left foot to the original position, eyes looking forward. Exhale while doing this.

Switch feet and do the same on the other side; repeat 6–8 times.

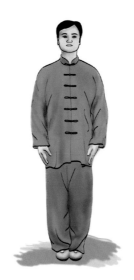

Key points

Turn the head to both sides to the same degree and at shoulder level. Avoid turning the spinal column, eyes looking as far back as possible.

Effect

This mainly adjusts the function of the central nervous system to improve the cervical vertebra, relax the cervical muscle, improve the oxygen and blood supply to the brain, and eliminate fatigue. Turn the waist to the sides to strengthen it and the kidneys, and to keep the spleen and stomach healthy. The movements can also be used to prevent hypertension, cervical vertebra problems, and eye trouble.

Note

It must be particularly noted that as the movements in this part require the turning of the head and neck, sufferers of cervical vertebra and dizziness should do the exercises with caution.

**V. Swinging the head and lowering the body
to relieve stress**

    Start by moving the left foot one step to the left. Bend
the knees to squat in a horse stance, and place the hands on
the knees, with the thumbs pointing backward, elbows bent,
eyes looking ahead.

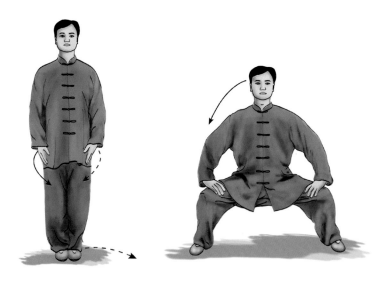

Bend the upper body low, forward and downward to the right as much as possible, so that the center of gravity falls on the right leg, and stretch the head forward as much as possible. Inhale while doing this exercise.

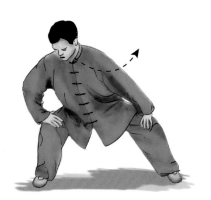

Bend the upper body low, and turn as far as possible to the left, wagging the buttocks; extend the right leg with the center of gravity shifting to the left leg, the buttocks wagging to the right, waist turned and hips in, eyes looking down to the right. Exhale while doing this exercise.

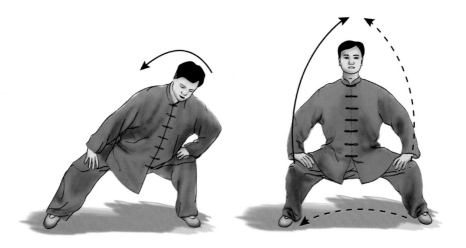

Turn the bent body to the right, wagging the buttocks, and do the same exercise as shown on page 72 but in the opposite direction. Move the hands in an arc from below upward, and drop them by the sides; draw the left foot back and return to the starting position.

Switch feet and do the same on the other side; repeat 6–8 times.

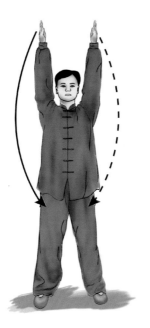
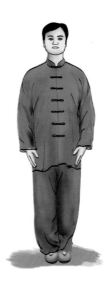

Key points

Be careful not to arch the back and drop the head. Bend the knees and turn the body equally to both sides; move the head and buttocks away from each other, with the waist stretched. Keep the hands on the knees, and the feet on the ground.

Effect

Wagging the head and the buttocks, and twisting the waist and hips helps to reduce the excitability of the central nervous system, eliminate heartburn, and calm the mind. At the same time, these movements help to improve the joints of the waist and neck, and prevent and cure diseases of the cervical vertebra and the abdominal vertebra, insomnia, heart palpitations, and nervousness.

Heartburn is an ailment caused by excessive internal fire in the organs.

Note

It must be particularly noted that as this part of the exercise requires the wagging of the head, neck, waist and buttocks together, sufferers of cervical vertebra and abdominal vertebra troubles should do the exercise with caution.

VI. Moving the hands down the back and legs, and touching the feet to strengthen the kidneys

Start by raising the hands to the top of the head in front of the body, palms up. Bend the upper body backward, keeping the head up. Inhale while doing this.

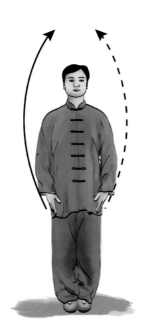 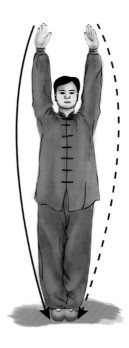

Move the hands downward to the toes while bending the upper body; use the fingers to hold the toes, knees extended. Exhale while doing this.

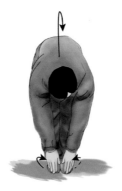

Raise the upper body, move the hands in an arc along the outer sides of the feet to the heels, and then upward along the back of the legs to the waist, both palms tightly against the muscles of the waist, fingertips down. Bend the upper body backward, head up. Inhale while doing this.

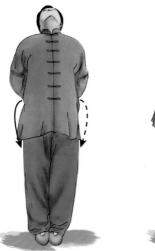
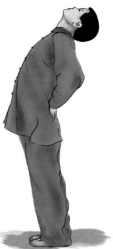

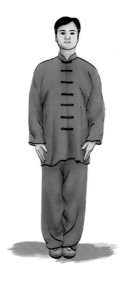

Move the hands downward naturally and return to the starting position. Exhale while doing this.

Key points

Don't bend back too far, just far enough to avoid incorrectly bending the waist and knees. Keep the knees straight all the time while bending forward or backward.

Repeat 6–8 times.

Effect

This exercise fully stretches the muscle groups of the waist and abdomen to draw the group of muscles at the back of the legs. This improves the pliability of the waist and legs, and prevents strain of the lumbar muscles and hip pain.

Note

It must be particularly noted that as it is difficult to hold the toes with both hands, sufferers of high blood pressure and hardening of the cerebral vessels should avoid bending forward too low, but do the exercise as their health allows.

VII. Thrusting the fists and making the eyes glare to enhance strength

Start by moving the left foot one big step to the left and bend the legs to squat in a horse stance. Clench the fists by the sides of the waist, palms up. Inhale while doing this.

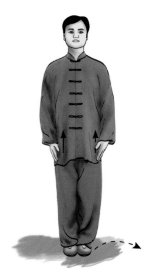 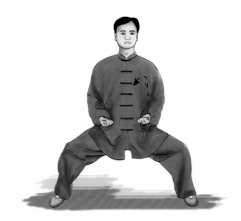

Punch the left fist forward, fist down, with the eyes wide open, and glare toward the left fist into the distance. Draw the right fist backward at the same time to make both arms compete with each other in pulling for power. Exhale while doing this.

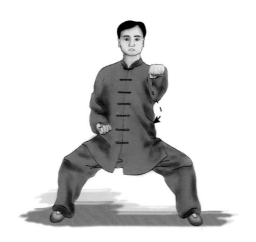

Move the left fist back to the left side of the waist; relax the hands and place palms by the sides of the body. At the same time, move the left foot back and return to the starting position.

Switch feet and do the same on the other side; repeat 6–8 times.

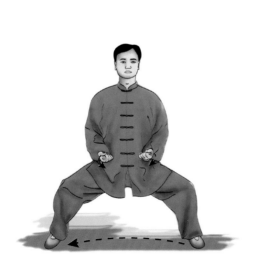
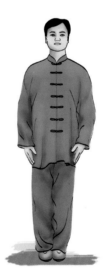

Key points

Don't raise the shoulders, hold waist too tightly or close the eyes. Relax the waist and sink the hips. Keep the shoulders and elbows down, with the *qi* flowing to the *dantian*. Exhaling and punching with angry eyes should occur simultaneously.

Glaring can stimulate the liver meridian and the passage of blood in the liver, thereby freeing up blocked *qi* in the liver and improving muscles and bones.

Effect

This is designed to improve the functions of the liver and regulate the *qi* and blood. Moreover, it also exercises the muscles of the back, limbs and eyes and strengthens the muscles and bones.

VIII. Raising and lowering the heels to cure diseases

Start by placing the hands on the abdomen, palms up and fingertips touching each other; move them up along the mid-torso to the front of the chest. Inhale while doing this.

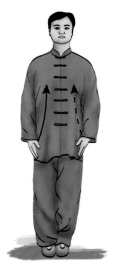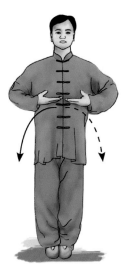

Turn the hands over, palms down and fingertips touching each other, and move them down along the mid-torso to the abdomen and then apart to both sides of the body, fingertips turned outside and forward, palms down. Exhale while doing this.

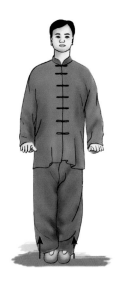

Keep the legs tightly together, straighten the legs and raise
the heels, head stretched up. Inhale while doing this.

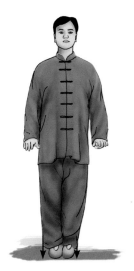 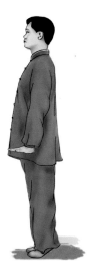

Shake the body naturally while putting the heels down.
Exhale while doing this. Repeat 6–8 times, and drop the
palms down and place them by the sides. The whole body
should be relaxed. Return to the starting position.

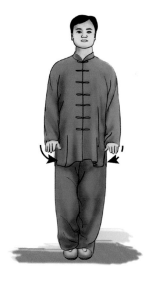
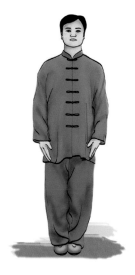

Key points

Make sure to keep balance while raising the heels. Keep the toes slightly apart, and shake slightly when putting the heels down. Relax the whole body.

Effect

This is the final part of the whole exercise, and it should be relaxing. Shake the body up and down rhythmically to temper the joints of the vertebrae and help to relax all the muscles of the body and the internal organs. This section is aimed at maintaining the smooth flow of *qi* and blood to help rid the body of disease.

Note

It must be particularly noted that people who have back problems should place on their heels down gently and refrain from exerting too much force.

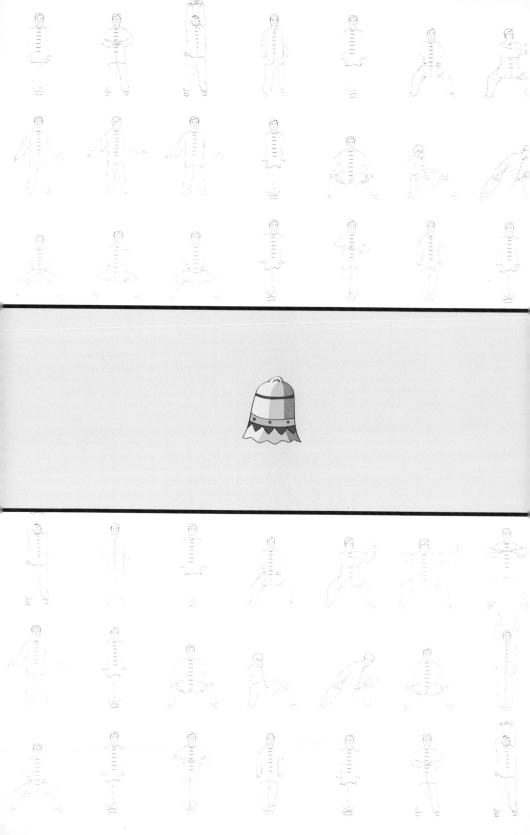

Points to Remember when Doing Qigong

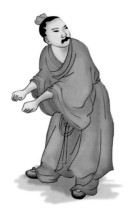

Five-animal Exercises—tiger

1. Stop all other sports and entertainment activities 30 minutes before starting *qigong* exercises. Be mentally prepared to do the exercises and free your mind from distractions. Be totally relaxed while doing the exercises. If you are irritable or have anything on your mind, don't do the exercises; wait until you can do them whole-heartedly.

2. Wear loose clothing when doing *qigong* exercises to facilitate the smooth circulation of the *qi* and blood. The color should be subdued and the cloth soft. Whether in the standing or lying posture, keep the belt and underwear loose so that breathing comes easily and blood flow is not hindered. Remove glasses, watches, headwear, jewelry or other ornaments.

3. In order to avoid stomach and intestine troubles, don't do the exercises if you are too hungry or too full. Defecate and urinate before doing the exercises. Drink some warm water before doing the exercise to improve blood circulation.

4. Choose a quiet and clean place to do your exercises. Whether outdoors or indoors, there should be soft light and fresh air; don't do the exercises in a drafty place. Generally speaking, the best place is in the woods, by a river and a hill.

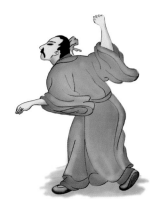

Five-animal Exercises—bear

5. Move your body in ways that you feel natural while doing the exercises. Don't thrust the chest out or raise the shoulders while in the standing, sitting or lying postures. Be sure your breathing is easy and natural. If the sitting posture is used, shake the upper body slightly after you are seated to get comfortable.

6. Do the closing move-ments well after you have

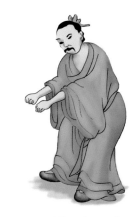

Five-animal Exercises—deer

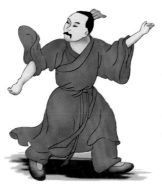

Five-animal Exercises—monkey

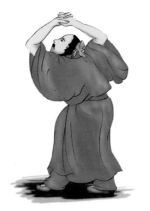

Five-animal Exercises—bird

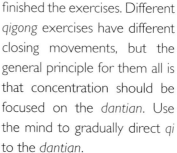

finished the exercises. Different *qigong* exercises have different closing movements, but the general principle for them all is that concentration should be focused on the *dantian*. Use the mind to gradually direct *qi* to the *dantian*.

7. Don't take a cold bath or wash your hands in cold water after doing *qigong* exercises. If you sweat, use a towel to wipe it off or take a warm bath.

8. Women should not do any exercises that involve concentrating on the *dantian*, abdominal breathing exercises or exercises requiring much physical exertion if they are menstruating, pregnant, or have just given birth. *Qigong* exercises should not be done during storms with thunder and lightning.

9. Do *qigong* exercises step by step and according to your capability; don't expect quick results. The effects of *qigong* exercise come from long-term practice. Moreover, different people should choose different exercises, depending on their body type and overall health.

10. Live a well-balanced life, keep a regular schedule for work and rest, and refrain from smoking and drinking; otherwise, even the most diligent practice of *qigong* won't be of any benefit.